Overcoming Weight Gain

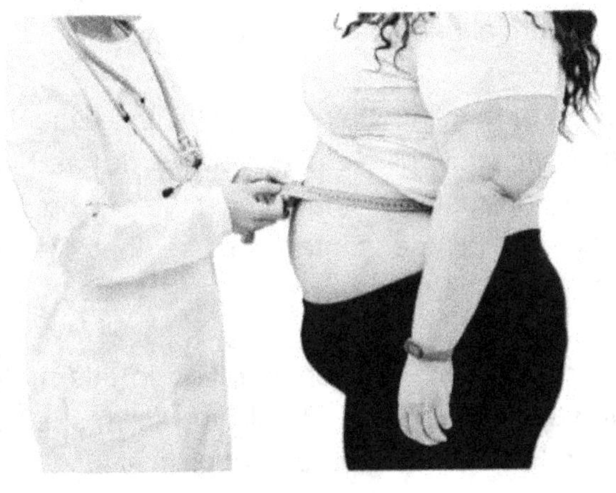

The A to Z Journey Towards Weight Loss

Dr Monique K. Roberts

Introduction

In the dimly lit hospital room, Sarah found herself at a crossroads. Tubes and monitors surrounded her, and the weight of her situation pressed heavily on her chest. She'd always been the caregiver, the rock for her family, but now, she lay frail, the result of years of neglecting her own well-being. The stark reality of her condition was an unwelcome wake-up call—a wake-up call that was long overdue.

Sarah's story is not unique. It's a tale shared by countless individuals who have faced the painful consequences of weight gain. The struggle with extra pounds had silently and insidiously taken control of her life until that fateful moment in the hospital room.

This book, "Overcoming Weight Gain," is not just another addition to the sea of weight loss guides. It's a lifeline. It's a bridge from where you are now to where you want to be. It's the culmination of wisdom gained from Sarah's journey, from the countless others who've fought the same battle, and from the experts who understand that this journey is about more than just shedding pounds.

But here's the truth that compelled me to write this book: Time is a fleeting commodity, and it's the one thing we can't afford to squander. Weight gain is more than just a physical burden; it can hold you back from the life you deserve. It can rob you of precious moments with loved ones, steal your energy, and undermine your confidence. It's time to take action.

The reason to read this book is simple: It's a call to action. Sarah's story is a reminder that time is finite, and the cost of inaction is too great. This book is your roadmap to reclaiming your health, rediscovering your confidence, and rewriting your own story of triumph.

In the pages ahead, you won't find empty promises or quick fixes. What you will find is a roadmap, a companion for your journey, and a testament to the power within you. This book is your chance to seize control, to script a new chapter in your life's story—one marked by determination, resilience, and ultimately, triumph.

Don't waste another moment. Your transformation begins with the turn of a page. Dive in, and let this book be your partner on the path to overcoming weight gain and embracing a life filled with health, vitality, and joy.. Weight gain is a deeply personal and sometimes painful journey, one that can feel like a relentless battle, testing not just our resolve but our self-worth. I know this struggle intimately, and I understand the tears of frustration, the longing for a healthier self, and the whispered dreams of a brighter tomorrow.

So, I implore you, don't waste another moment. The reasons to embark on this journey are countless—your health, your happiness, your future. With every page you turn, you move one step closer to overcoming weight gain and embracing the life you've yearned for. It's not a matter of if, but when, you'll experience the transformation you so deeply desire.

Let's begin this transformative journey together. Your better tomorrow starts right here, right now.

Table of Contents

Chapter 1: Understanding Weight Gain

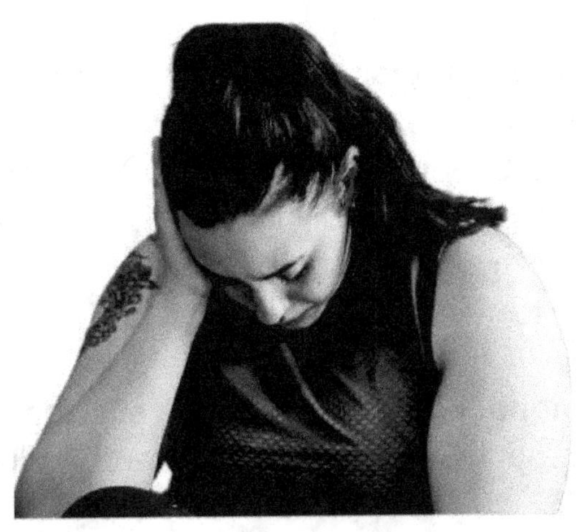

Weight gain is a complex and multifaceted phenomenon that touches the lives of millions worldwide. It's a topic that goes beyond the superficial concern of appearance, delving deep into the realms of biology, genetics, psychology, and lifestyle. To truly conquer weight gain, we must first embark on a journey of understanding. In this comprehensive exploration, we unravel the intricacies of weight gain, peeling back the layers to reveal the profound insights it holds.

The Basics of Weight Gain: At its core, weight gain is a simple equation: when we consume more calories than our bodies burn, the excess is stored as fat, leading to weight gain. This is a fundamental principle that underscores the importance of maintaining a caloric balance.

Genetic Predisposition: Genetics play a significant role in determining an individual's susceptibility to weight gain. Some people may have a genetic predisposition to store calories as fat more efficiently, making them more prone to gaining weight.

Hormonal Factors: Hormones such as insulin, leptin, and ghrelin exert powerful influences over our appetite and metabolism. Understanding how these hormones work and how imbalances can lead to weight gain is crucial for managing one's weight effectively.

Psychological Aspects: Emotional and psychological factors often contribute to weight gain. Emotional stress, unhealthy eating habits, and mental well-being can disturb our diet and result in excessive calorie intake.

Environmental Factors: The environment we live in, characterized by the availability of calorie-dense foods and sedentary lifestyles, can promote weight gain. An obesogenic environment poses significant challenges to maintaining a healthy weight.

Metabolism: Metabolism, the body's energy-burning process, varies from person to person. Some individuals have a higher metabolism and can burn calories more efficiently, while others have a slower metabolism, making it easier for them to gain weight.

Inflammation and Weight Gain: Chronic inflammation, often a result of poor dietary choices and a sedentary lifestyle, has been linked to weight gain and obesity. This inflammatory state can disrupt normal metabolic processes.

Health Consequences: Weight gain is not just about aesthetics; it's about health. Excess weight can lead to a host of health issues, including type 2 diabetes, heart disease, and certain cancers. Recognizing these health consequences underscores the importance of addressing weight gain proactively.

To truly overcome weight gain, one must embrace a holistic understanding of this multifaceted issue. It's not just about reducing caloric intake or increasing physical activity; it's about addressing the genetic, hormonal, psychological, and environmental factors that contribute to it. Armed with this comprehensive knowledge, individuals can approach their weight loss journey with informed strategies and a better chance of achieving lasting success.

Understanding weight gain is the first step towards transformation, leading to a healthier, more vibrant life. It empowers individuals to make choices that promote wellness and enables them to navigate the challenges and complexities of weight management with wisdom and resilience.

Chapter 2: The Science Behind Weight Gain

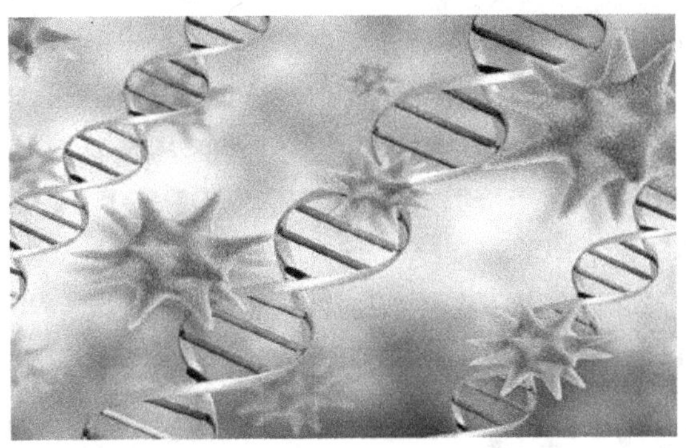

Certainly! Weight gain is a complex process influenced by various factors, and understanding the science behind it is essential for maintaining a healthy lifestyle. This note will delve into the key components of weight gain and provide insights into the physiological and environmental factors at play.

Caloric Balance: The fundamental principle of weight gain is the balance between calorie intake and expenditure. When you consume more calories than your body needs for daily activities and metabolic functions, the excess calories are stored as fat, leading to weight gain. Conversely, if you consume fewer calories than your body expends, weight loss occurs. The calorie balance equation is at the core of weight management.

Metabolism: Metabolism plays a pivotal role in weight gain. It refers to the processes by which your body converts food into energy and manages the use of that energy. Basal metabolic rate (BMR) is the energy your body requires to maintain basic functions at rest. Factors such as genetics, age, and muscle mass influence your BMR. People with a higher BMR burn more calories even when they're not active, making it easier for them to maintain or lose weight.

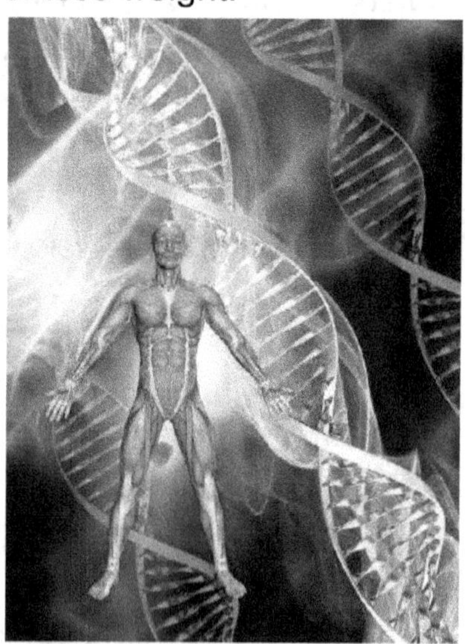

Nutrient Quality: It's not just about the quantity of calories; the quality of the nutrients matters as well. Highly processed and sugary foods can lead to weight gain because they are often calorie-dense but nutrient-poor. In contrast, whole, unprocessed foods provide essential nutrients and fiber, promoting feelings of fullness and aiding in weight control.

Hormonal Regulation: Hormones like insulin, leptin, and ghrelin play a crucial role in regulating hunger and satiety. Insulin is released in response to blood sugar levels and promotes fat storage, while leptin signals fullness to the brain. Ghrelin, on the other hand, stimulates hunger. Hormonal imbalances or insensitivity can disrupt these signals, contributing to weight gain.

Psychological Factors: Emotional and psychological factors can significantly impact weight gain. Emotional overeating often results from stress, boredom, and calorie surplus. Moreover, individual behaviors, like eating habits, portion sizes, and frequency of meals, can affect the overall caloric intake.

Physical Activity: Physical activity, including both exercise and daily movement, plays a vital role in weight management. Regular exercise not only burns calories but also builds lean muscle mass, which increases your BMR. Sedentary lifestyles can lead to weight gain as calorie expenditure decreases.

Environmental Influences: The obesogenic environment, characterized by the ready availability of high-calorie, low-nutrient foods, and sedentary activities, is a significant contributor to weight gain. Access to unhealthy foods and reduced opportunities for physical activity can make weight gain more likely.

In conclusion, weight gain is a multifaceted process influenced by caloric balance, metabolism, nutrient quality, hormonal regulation, psychological factors, physical activity, and environmental influences. Understanding these factors is essential for managing and maintaining a healthy weight.

Achieving and sustaining a healthy weight involves adopting a balanced diet, staying physically active, and being mindful of the psychological and environmental influences on your choices. It's important to consult with healthcare professionals and nutrition experts to develop a personalized and sustainable plan for managing weight.

Chapter 3: Types of Weight Gain: Is There More Than One?

Certainly! Weight gain can be categorized into several types, each with distinct causes and implications. Understanding these types of weight gain is crucial for addressing the underlying issues and developing appropriate strategies for weight management. Here are some common types of weight gain:

1. Normal/Physiological Weight Gain:

This type of weight gain is a natural part of life and occurs during various life stages. Examples include:

Infant Growth: Babies naturally gain weight as they grow, and it's essential for their development.

Adolescence: Adolescents often experience growth spurts and gain weight as they mature.

Pregnancy: Weight gain during pregnancy is necessary for the health of the mother and the developing fetus.

2. Overnutrition-Related Weight Gain:

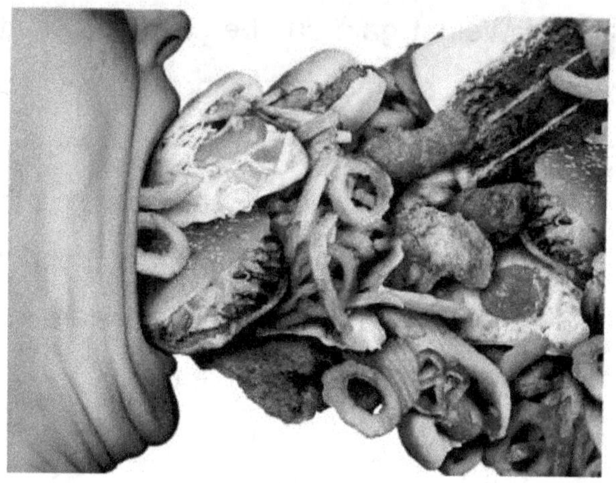

Overnutrition occurs when individuals consistently consume more calories than their bodies require. This type of weight gain is often associated with poor dietary choices and a sedentary lifestyle. It can lead to overweight and obesity, and may result from:

Excessive Caloric Intake: Consuming more calories than the body can burn leads to weight gain.

Unhealthy Diet: Diets high in processed foods, sugary beverages, and saturated fats contribute to overnutrition-related weight gain.

Sedentary Lifestyle: Lack of physical activity can hinder calorie expenditure.

3. Hormonally-Induced Weight Gain:

Hormones play a crucial role in regulating weight, and imbalances can lead to weight gain. Some hormonal conditions include:

Hypothyroidism: A sluggish thyroid can lead to reduced metabolism and weight gain.

Polycystic Ovary Syndrome (PCOS): PCOS is associated with hormonal imbalances that can cause weight gain, particularly in the abdominal area.

Cushing's Syndrome: An excess of cortisol, often due to medical conditions or medications, can lead to weight gain.

4. Medication-Induced Weight Gain:

Certain medications, including antidepressants, antipsychotics, and corticosteroids, may cause weight gain as a side effect. This weight gain is not related to overnutrition but can be challenging to manage.

5. Stress-Related Weight Gain:

Chronic stress can lead to weight gain in some individuals. The release of stress hormones, such as cortisol, can increase appetite and promote fat storage, particularly in the abdominal area.

6. Fluid Retention Weight Gain:

Temporary weight gain can occur due to water retention, often linked to various factors, including:

Sodium Intake: High sodium intake can cause the body to retain excess water.

Menstrual Cycle: Some women experience water retention during their menstrual cycle.

Medical Conditions: Conditions like edema can cause fluid retention and temporary weight gain.

7. Muscle Mass Gain:

Weight gain from an increase in muscle mass is a positive type of weight gain. It is often seen in individuals engaged in strength training or resistance exercises. Muscle weighs more than fat, so building muscle can lead to an increase in body weight while improving body composition.

8. Aging-Related Weight Gain:

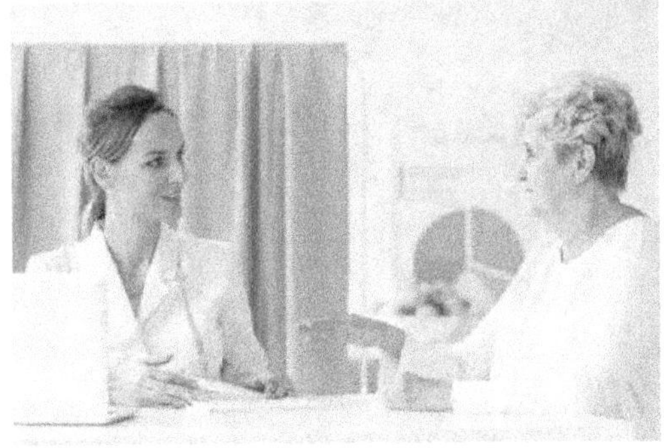

As people age, their metabolism tends to slow down, and they may become less active.

These factors can contribute to gradual weight gain over time.

Understanding the type of weight gain you're experiencing is essential for devising an effective approach to address it. Consultation with a healthcare professional or a registered dietitian can help you identify the underlying causes and develop a personalized plan for weight management, whether it involves dietary changes, increased physical activity, hormone management, or stress reduction strategies.

Chapter 4: The Role of Genetics

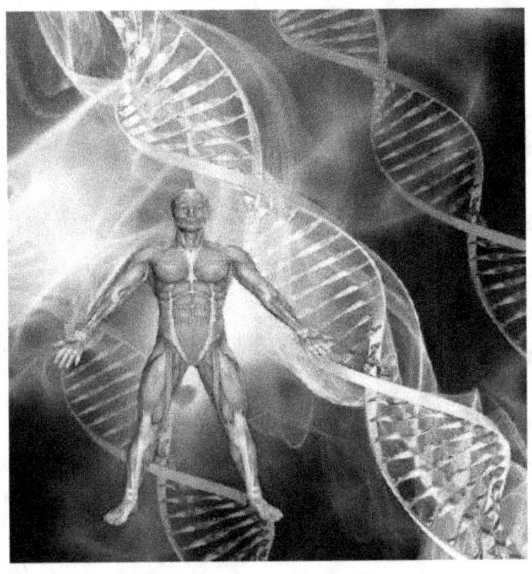

Certainly! The role of genetics in weight gain is a complex and multifaceted topic. While genetics can influence various aspects of an individual's body composition and metabolism, it's essential to recognize that genetics is just one piece of the puzzle. Here's an elaborate look at how genetics can play a role in weight gain:

1. Genetic Predisposition:

Body Type: Genes contribute to an individual's body type, which can influence how fat is distributed. Some people may be genetically predisposed to store fat in specific areas, such as the abdomen or hips, which can affect overall body weight and shape.

Metabolism: Genetics can influence an individual's basal metabolic rate (BMR), which is the number of calories the body burns at rest. Some people may inherit a faster metabolism, making it easier to maintain a healthy weight, while others may have a slower metabolism, which can contribute to weight gain if not managed carefully.

2. Appetite Regulation:

Leptin and Ghrelin: Genetic variations can impact the regulation of hormones like leptin and ghrelin, which play a critical role in appetite control. An individual's genetic makeup can influence how these hormones signal hunger

and satiety, making some people more prone
to overeating.

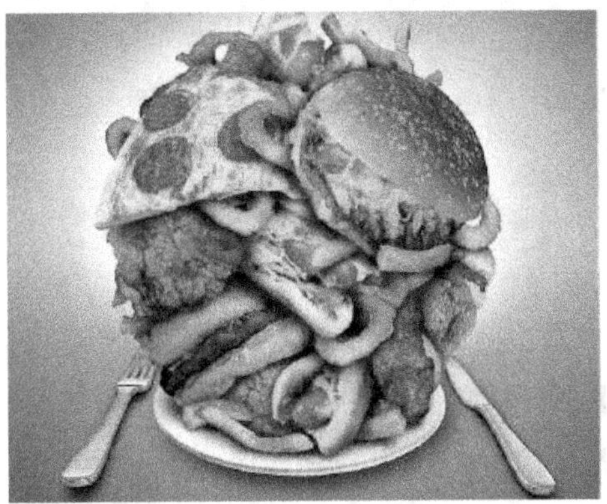

Taste Preferences: Genetic factors can
influence taste preferences, affecting an
individual's inclination toward sweet, salty, or
fatty foods. These preferences can impact
dietary choices and, in turn, weight gain.

3. Obesity-Related Genes:

FTO Gene: The FTO gene is often referred to
as the "fat mass and obesity-associated gene."
Variations in this gene have been associated
with an increased risk of obesity. It can affect
appetite and food intake, making individuals

with certain FTO gene variants more susceptible to weight gain.

MC4R Gene: Mutations in the MC4R gene are linked to the regulation of appetite and energy expenditure. Defects in this gene can lead to overeating and obesity in affected individuals.

4. Response to Diet and Exercise:

Genetic factors can influence how an individual responds to dietary changes and exercise:

Nutrigenetics: This field studies how genetics affects an individual's response to different diets. Some people may benefit more from low-carb diets, while others may respond better to low-fat diets based on their genetic makeup.

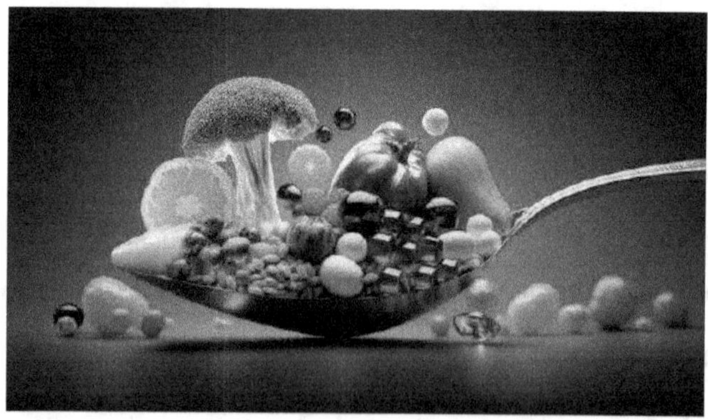

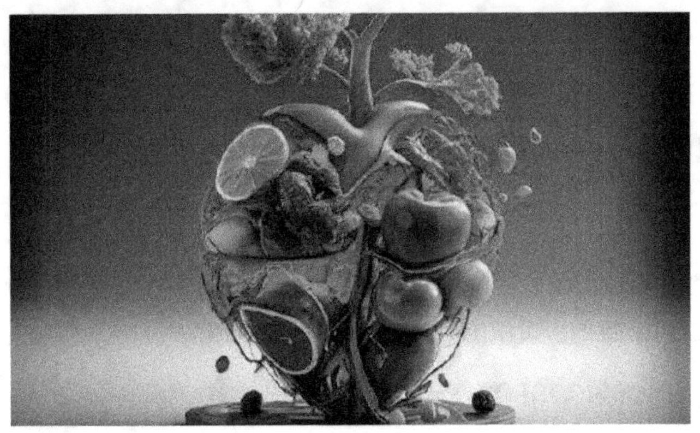

Exercise Genetics: Genetic variations can impact how efficiently a person's body burns calories during exercise. Some individuals may have a genetic advantage in terms of building lean muscle mass or burning fat through physical activity.

It's important to note that genetics is not the sole determinant of weight gain. Environmental factors, such as diet, physical activity, stress, and access to unhealthy foods, also play a significant role. Most importantly, genetics should not be used as an excuse for unhealthy habits. While genetics can create a predisposition to weight gain, lifestyle choices and behavior modifications remain essential in managing weight effectively.

Individuals interested in understanding their genetic predisposition to weight gain can consider genetic testing, but it's important to do so in consultation with a healthcare professional or genetic counselor. A personalized approach that combines genetic insights with healthy lifestyle choices is often the most effective strategy for maintaining a healthy weight.

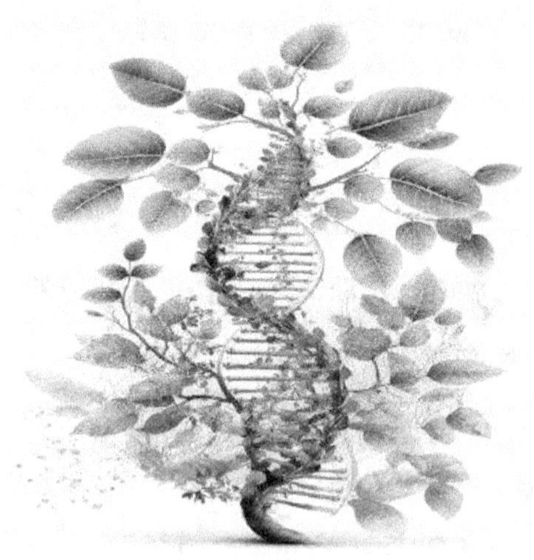

Chapter 5: The Impact of Lifestyle and Environment

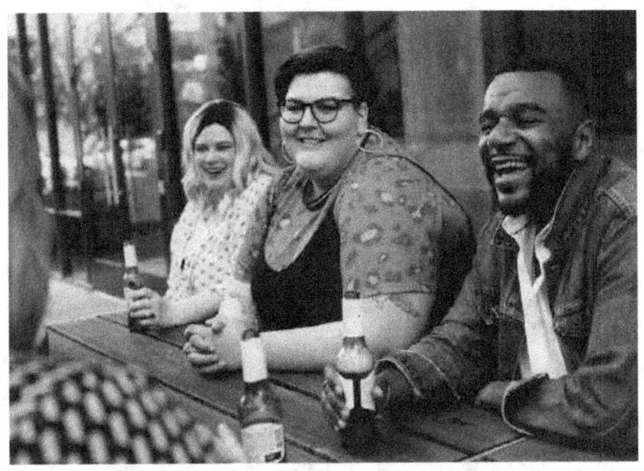

The impact of lifestyle and environment on weight gain is profound and multifaceted. Various factors within one's daily life and surroundings can significantly influence body weight and, by extension, overall health. Here's an elaborate and comprehensive exploration of this complex relationship:

1. Dietary Habits:

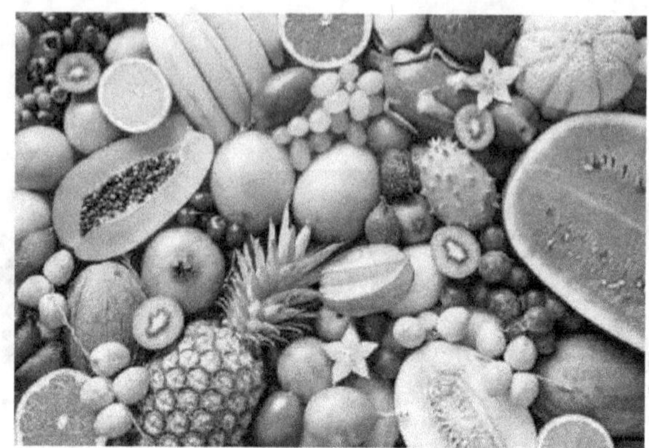

Food Choices: The types of foods individuals choose to consume can greatly impact weight. A diet rich in whole, unprocessed foods, including fruits, vegetables, lean proteins, and whole grains, tends to support a healthy weight. In contrast, diets high in processed, sugary, and high-fat foods can contribute to weight gain.

Portion Sizes: Large portion sizes can lead to overconsumption of calories. Super-sized meals and oversized servings in restaurants can encourage excessive calorie intake.

__Eating Patterns__: Irregular eating patterns, such as skipping meals or late-night eating, can disrupt the body's metabolism and lead to weight gain.

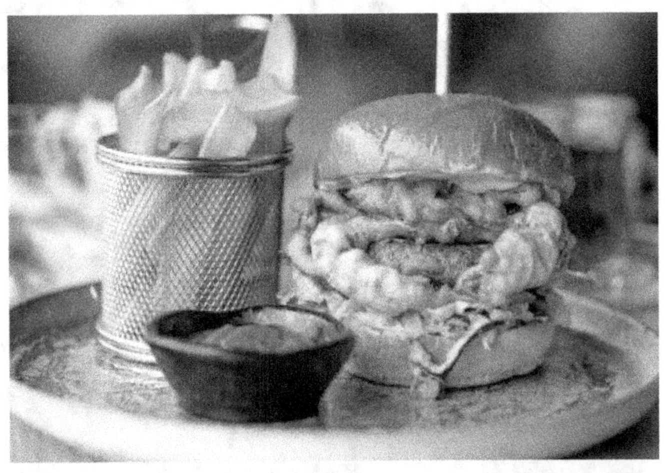

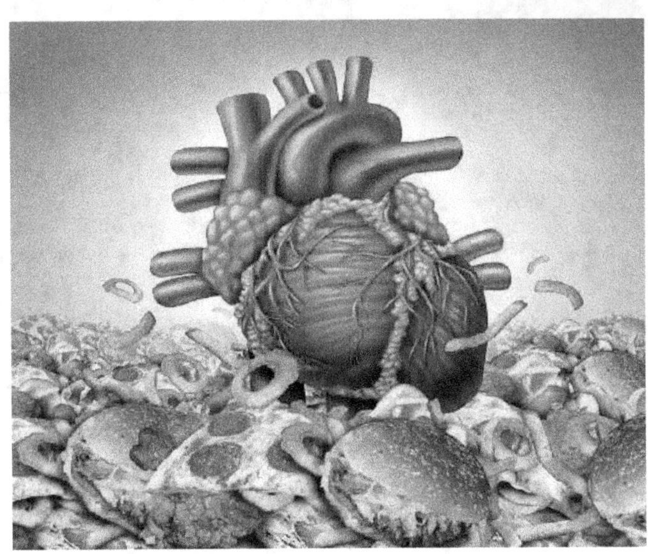

2. Physical Activity:

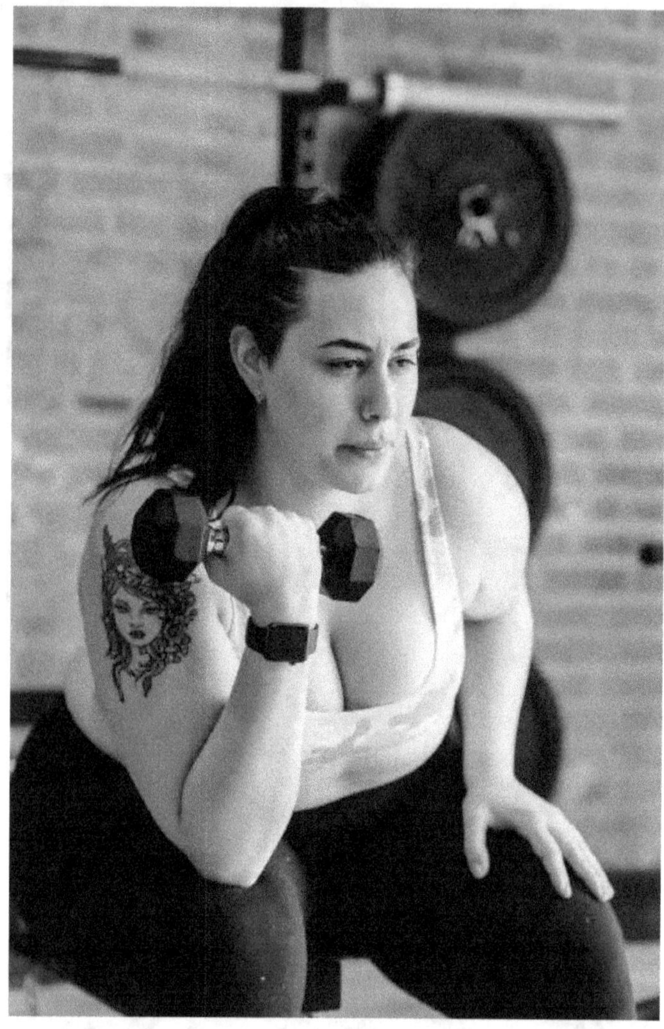

Sedentary Lifestyle: A lack of physical activity can be a significant contributor to weight gain. Many modern jobs and leisure activities involve sitting for extended periods, reducing calorie expenditure.

Exercise: Regular physical activity, including cardiovascular exercise, strength training, and flexibility exercises, can help burn calories, build muscle, and support weight management.

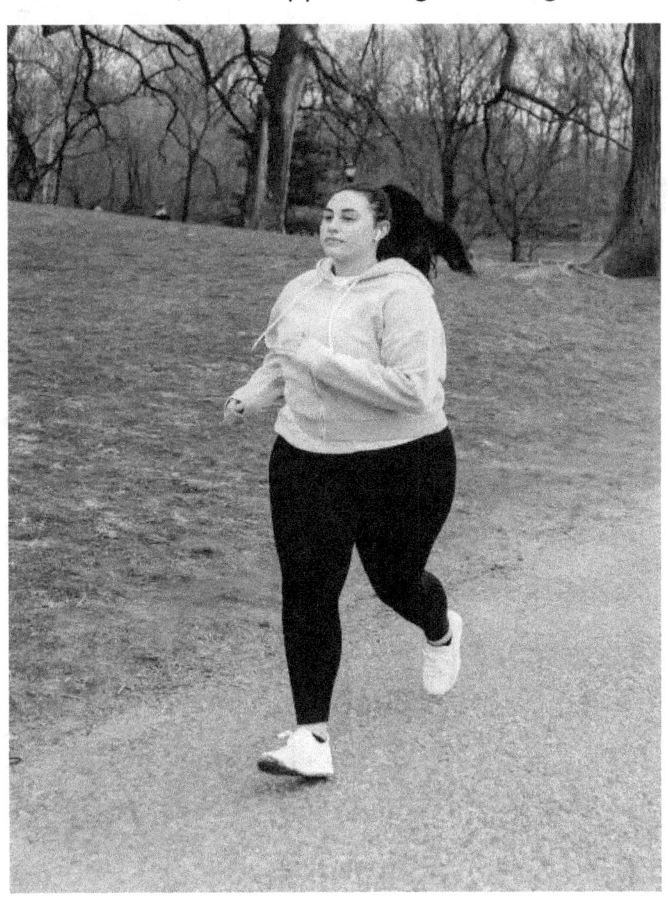

3. Socioeconomic Factors:

Access to Healthy Foods: Socioeconomic status can affect access to affordable, nutritious foods. Lower-income individuals often have limited access to fresh produce and healthy food options, which can lead to reliance on cheaper, less nutritious alternatives.

Education: Understanding nutrition and health plays a crucial role. Lack of nutrition education can lead to poor dietary choices and contribute to weight gain.

4. Psychological Factors:

Stress: Persistent stress may trigger emotional eating, causing high-calorie cravings and weight gain due to overindulgence in comfort foods.

Mental Health: Conditions such as depression and anxiety can be associated with changes in appetite and weight. Weight gain is a potential side effect of medications used for these conditions.

5. Food Environment:

Food Marketing: Extensive marketing of high-calorie, low-nutrient foods can influence dietary choices. Advertisements for unhealthy products and promotions can encourage overconsumption.

Food Availability: The ready availability of fast food, convenience stores, and vending machines with unhealthy options can make it challenging to maintain a healthy diet.

6. Social and Cultural Influences:

Social Norms: Eating behaviors within a person's social and cultural context can impact weight gain. Social gatherings and celebrations often revolve around food, potentially leading to overeating.

Family and Peer Influence: The eating habits and lifestyle choices of family members and peers can influence an individual's own behavior.

7. Built Environment:

Walkability: Communities designed for walking and physical activity can encourage more movement, while car-dependent environments may discourage physical activity.

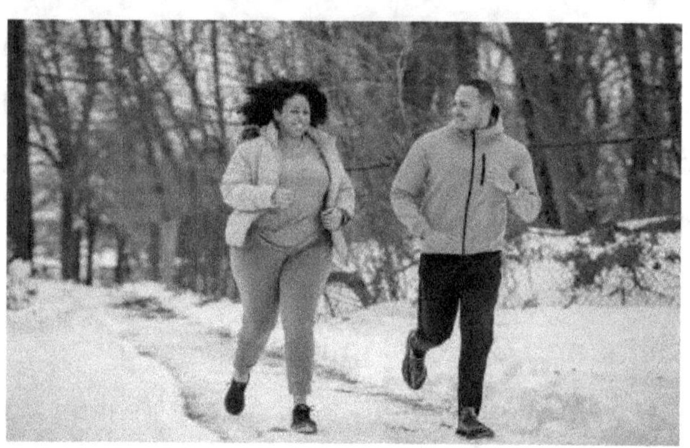

Access to Recreational Facilities: The availability of parks, gyms, and recreational facilities can affect an individual's ability to engage in physical activity.

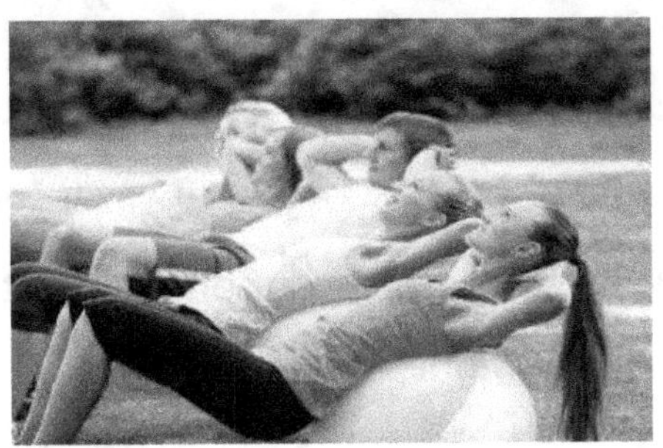

8. Sleep Patterns:

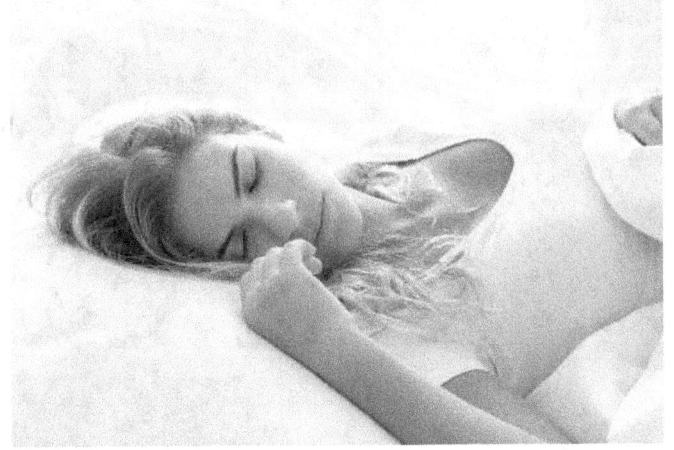

Sleep Duration: Inadequate sleep can disrupt hormonal regulation, affecting hunger and appetite. People who consistently get insufficient sleep may be at higher risk of weight gain.

9. Environmental Toxins:

Endocrine Disruptors: Certain environmental toxins, such as some chemicals in plastics and pesticides, can disrupt hormonal regulation and potentially contribute to weight gain.

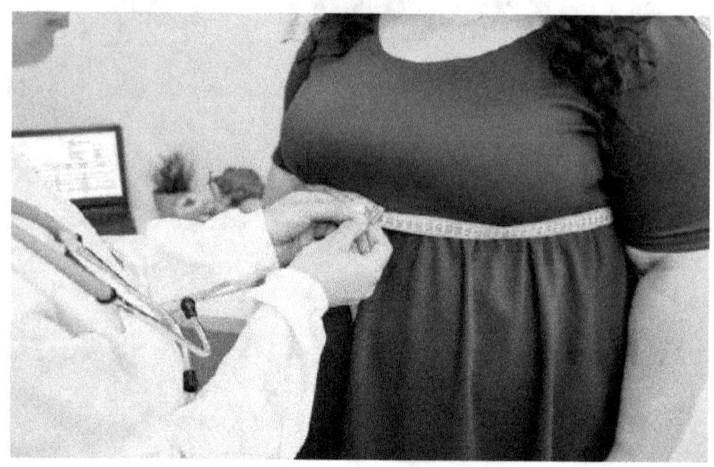

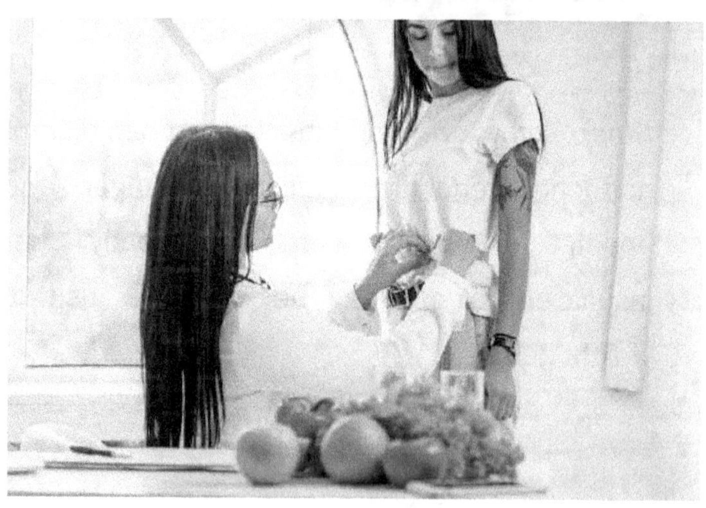

Chapter 6: Emotional Eating: The Hidden Culprit

Emotional eating is a significant but often overlooked factor contributing to weight gain and unhealthy eating habits. It involves using food as a means to cope with emotional distress, stress, boredom, or other feelings. This comprehensive content delves into the phenomenon of emotional eating, its underlying causes, consequences, and strategies to overcome it.

Emotional eating, also known as stress eating or comfort eating, refers to the practice of consuming food not out of physical hunger but to soothe or suppress emotional issues. These emotions can include stress, anxiety, sadness, loneliness, boredom, anger, or even happiness. It's essential to understand that occasional emotional eating is a normal human response, but when it becomes a habitual and uncontrollable pattern, it can have adverse effects on physical and mental health.

Causes of Emotional Eating:

1. Stress and Coping: Stress is one of the most common triggers for emotional eating. The release of stress hormones can lead to cravings for high-calorie, comfort foods, as the brain seeks a quick dopamine release for relaxation.

2. Emotional Regulation: Food can act as a temporary mood enhancer. Eating can provide a sense of comfort and emotional relief, which some individuals seek when dealing with negative emotions.

3. Boredom: Monotony and boredom can lead to eating for entertainment. This type of eating is often unplanned and may involve snacking on unhealthy foods simply to pass the time.

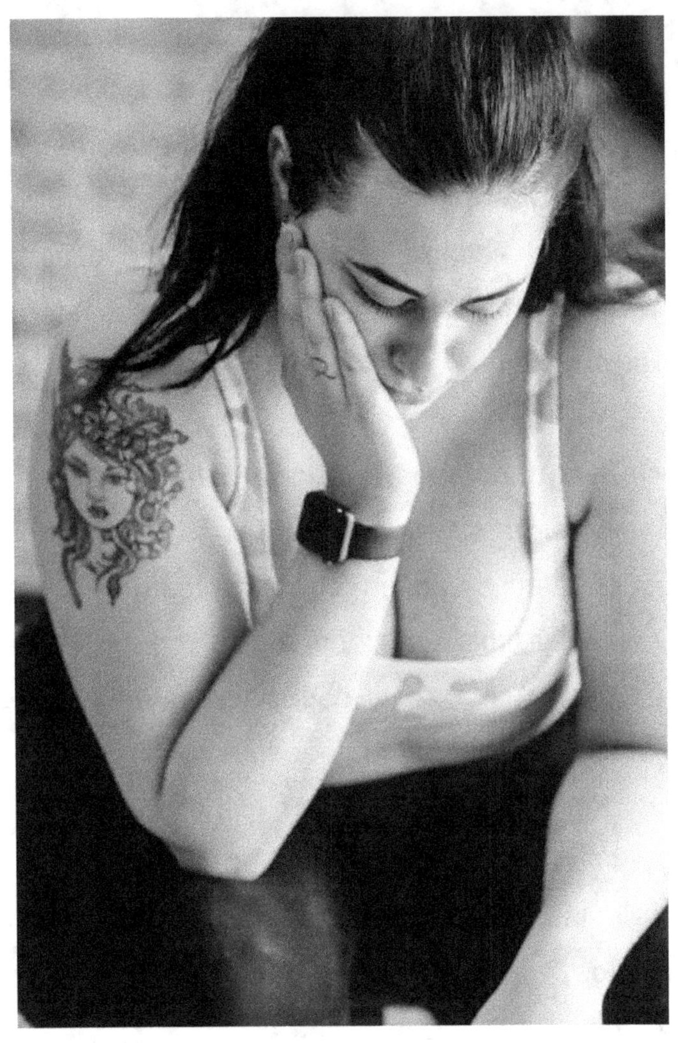

4. *Social and Cultural Influences*: Social gatherings, celebrations, and cultural norms often revolve around food, which can encourage overeating, even when emotional triggers are not present.

5. _Negative Self-Image_: Low self-esteem and body dissatisfaction can contribute to emotional eating. People may use food as a way to numb their feelings of inadequacy or to reward themselves when they feel unworthy.

Consequences of Emotional Eating

1. _Weight Gain:_ The consumption of calorie-dense comfort foods can lead to weight gain over time. Emotional eating is often linked to overconsumption, especially of unhealthy, high-sugar, and high-fat foods.

2. _Psychological Impact_: Emotional eating can create a cycle of guilt, shame, and self-blame. This can exacerbate the emotional issues that triggered the eating in the first place.

3. _Physical Health Implications_: Overeating and weight gain resulting from emotional eating can contribute to a range of health problems, including obesity, diabetes, and heart disease.

4. *Mental Health Issues*: Emotional eating is linked to a higher risk of mental health conditions, such as depression, anxiety, and eating disorders.

Strategies to Overcome Emotional Eating

1. *Mindful Eating*: Practicing mindfulness can help individuals become more aware of their eating habits and emotional triggers. Mindful eating involves paying close attention to the taste, texture, and sensations of food, helping to distinguish true hunger from emotional eating.

2. *Emotional Awareness*: Identifying and acknowledging the emotions that trigger eating is a crucial step. Finding alternative, healthier coping mechanisms for stress, boredom, and other emotional issues is essential.

3. *Stress Management*: Incorporating stress-reduction techniques, such as meditation, yoga, or deep breathing exercises, can help manage stress without turning to food for comfort.

4. Seeking Support: Talking to a therapist, counselor, or a support group can provide valuable insights and guidance for addressing emotional eating.

5. Healthy Food Choices: Stocking the kitchen with nutritious foods and avoiding the purchase of comfort foods can reduce the likelihood of overindulging.

6. Establishing Regular Meal Times: Eating at regular intervals can help prevent impulsive snacking due to boredom or emotional triggers.

In Conclusion, emotional eating is a hidden culprit behind weight gain and can have profound consequences on physical and mental health. Recognizing emotional eating patterns, understanding the underlying causes, and implementing strategies to manage emotional triggers is crucial for breaking the cycle and fostering healthier eating habits.

Chapter 7: The Mind-Body Connection

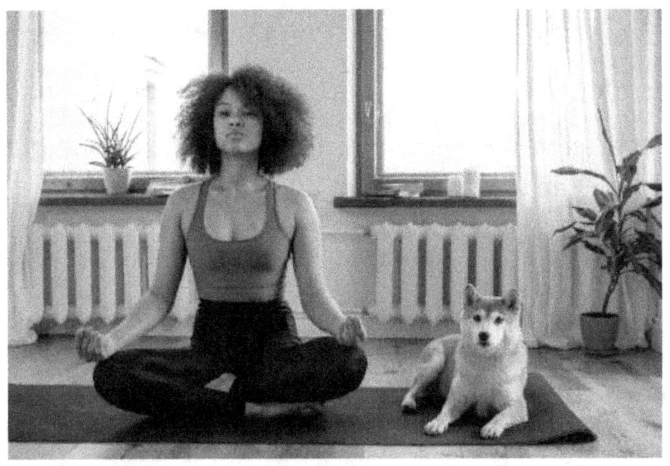

The mind-body connection is a powerful and intricate aspect of weight gain, with mental and emotional factors significantly influencing an individual's body weight. Note that the interplay between the mind and body in the context of weight gain, highlighting the psychological, emotional, and behavioral aspects can lead to increased body weight where there are strategies to harness this connection for effective weight management.

The mind-body connection encompasses the profound relationship between an individual's mental and emotional states and their physical health. It underscores the idea that one's thoughts, emotions, and behaviors can profoundly impact the body's functions and overall well-being. In the context of weight gain, this connection reveals that various mental and emotional factors can be key contributors to changes in body weight.

Psychological and Emotional Factors in Weight Gain

1. Stress and Emotional Eating:Chronic stress can trigger emotional eating, wherein individuals consume high-calorie comfort foods as a response to stress, anxiety, or emotional distress. Stress hormones like cortisol can lead to cravings for such foods, contributing to weight gain over time.

2. Depression and Weight Gain: Depression can lead to changes in appetite, often resulting in overeating or, conversely, loss of appetite. Weight gain can be a common side effect of depression and can further exacerbate the condition.

3. *Comfort Eating*: People sometimes turn to food as a source of comfort and emotional relief. The emotional bond with eating may result in excessive calorie-rich food intake, contributing to increased body weight.

4. *Self-Esteem and Body Image*: Low self-esteem and a negative body image can impact an individual's relationship with food and exercise. Some may use food as a way to cope with feelings of inadequacy or as a reward to compensate for a perceived lack of self-worth.

Behavioral Aspects in Weight Gain

1. *Binge Eating*: Binge eating disorder is characterized by consuming large quantities of food in a short time, often accompanied by feelings of loss of control. This behavior can lead to significant weight gain.

2. Eating Habits: Unhealthy eating habits such as frequent snacking, late-night eating, and irregular meal patterns can disrupt the body's metabolism and lead to overeating.

Strategies for Utilizing the Mind-Body Connection for Weight Management

1. Stress Management: Adopt stress-reduction techniques like meditation, deep breathing exercises, and yoga to manage stress effectively and reduce emotional eating.

2. Emotional Awareness: Identifying and acknowledging emotional triggers for overeating is crucial. Developing alternative, healthier coping mechanisms for emotional distress is essential for weight management.

3. Mindful Eating: Practice mindfulness during meals, paying attention to the sensory aspects of eating. It aids in distinguishing genuine hunger from emotional eating effectively.

4. *Support and Therapy*: Seek support from therapists, counselors, or support groups to address emotional factors contributing to weight gain. Cognitive-behavioral therapy can be particularly effective in addressing emotional eating.

5. *Self-Compassion*: Practice self-compassion to reduce self-criticism and guilt associated with overeating. A kind and understanding attitude toward oneself can promote healthier eating behaviors.

6. *Healthy Lifestyle Choices*: Adopt a holistic approach to health that includes regular physical activity and a balanced, nutritious diet. Focusing on long-term well-being rather than short-term weight loss can promote a positive relationship with one's body.

Therefore, the mind-body connection plays a significant role in weight gain, with mental and emotional factors often contributing to unhealthy eating habits and lifestyle choices. By recognizing the profound influence of the mind on the body, individuals can take steps to manage stress, cope with emotions more effectively, and develop healthier relationships with food. Harnessing the mind-body connection is a key aspect of successful weight management and overall well-being, promoting not just weight loss but also a healthier and more balanced life.

Chapter 8: Preparing for Change

Preparation for weight loss is a crucial step on the path to achieving and maintaining a healthier body weight. Effective weight loss requires a thoughtful, informed, and comprehensive approach. Here is a well-explained note on how to prepare for a successful weight loss journey:

1. Set Clear and Realistic Goals:

Start with setting realistic weight loss objectives for clarity and attainability. Consider how much weight you want to lose, your desired timeline, and the reasons behind your weight loss objectives. Realistic goals provide a sense of purpose and motivation.

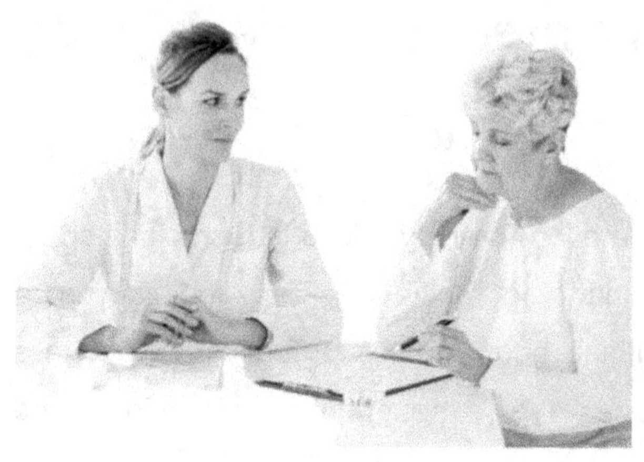

2. Consult with Healthcare Professionals:

Before embarking on any weight loss journey, it's advisable to consult with a healthcare provider or a registered dietitian. They can assess your current health status, identify any underlying medical conditions, and provide personalized guidance for your weight loss plan. By consulting healthcare professionals, they help you determine a healthy weight range, and identify any underlying medical conditions that may affect your goals.

3. Self-Education:

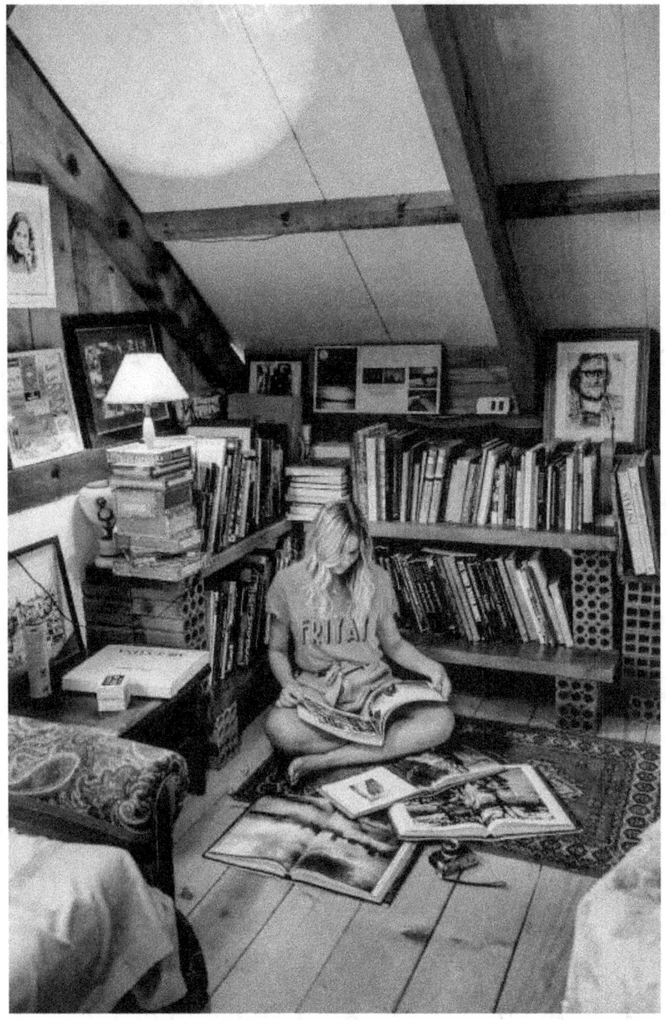

Educate yourself about nutrition, exercise, and

weight management. Understanding the basics

of calories, macronutrients, and the impact of

various foods on your body can help you make informed choices.

4. Create a Balanced Diet:

Develop a sustainable and balanced diet plan. Prioritize whole, natural foods like fruits, veggies, lean proteins, whole grains, and beneficial fats in your diet. Strive for a diet that provides essential nutrients while maintaining a calorie deficit for weight loss.

5. Portion Control:

Pay attention to portion sizes to avoid overeating. Using smaller plates, measuring portions, and practicing mindful eating can help you manage your food intake.

6. Plan Your Meals:

Plan your meals and snacks in advance. This can prevent impulsive, unhealthy choices and help you maintain a consistent eating schedule.

7. Regular Physical Activity:

Incorporate regular physical activity into your routine. Strive for a mix of cardio, strength workouts, and flexibility routines. Maintaining consistency is crucial for effective weight loss.

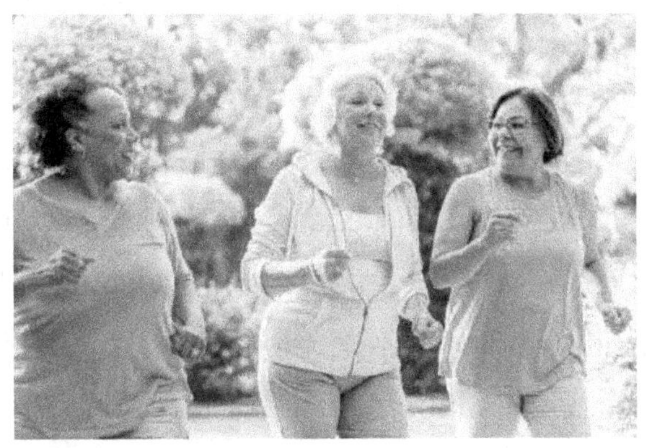

8. Keep a Food Journal:

Track your food intake to monitor your eating habits and identify areas for improvement. A food journal can also help you stay accountable and recognize patterns in your eating behaviors.

9. Mindful Eating:

Practice mindful eating by being fully present during meals, savoring the flavors, and recognizing your body's hunger and fullness cues. It helps avoid overindulgence and encourages better food selection.

10. Support System:

Build a support network. Share your weight loss goals with friends and family who can provide encouragement and accountability. Consider joining a weight loss group or seeking professional support if needed.

11. Manage Emotional Triggers:

Recognize emotional cues for excessive eating and establish alternative coping strategies. Stress management techniques, like meditation or relaxation exercises, can help.

12. Celebrate Small Wins:

Acknowledge and rejoice in your advancement, including minor milestones on your journey.. Positive reinforcement can help maintain motivation.

13. Stay Hydrated:

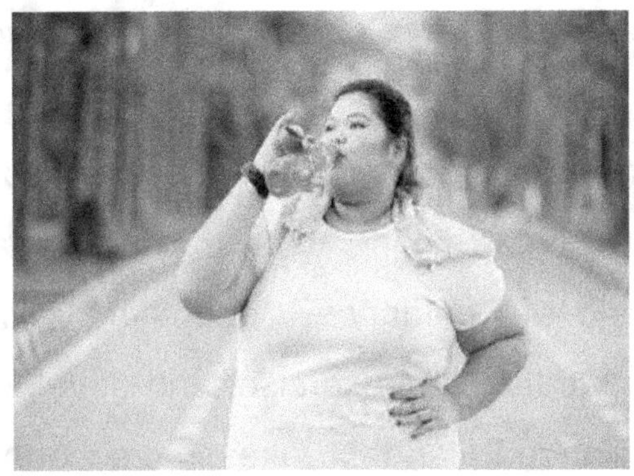

Drinking enough water is essential for weight loss. At times, thirst is confused with hunger, resulting in needless calorie intake.

14. Be Patient:

Understand that successful weight loss takes time and effort. It's a gradual process, and there may be plateaus or setbacks. Stay patient and persistent.

15. Regular Check-Ins:

Schedule regular check-ins with your healthcare provider or dietitian to monitor your progress, adjust your plan as needed, and ensure that you're losing weight in a healthy and sustainable way.

So, preparing for weight loss is a critical step that involves setting clear goals, obtaining professional guidance, educating yourself about nutrition and exercise, and developing a well-balanced plan that takes into account your unique needs and circumstances. By following these steps and approaching weight loss with a realistic, sustainable mindset, you can increase your chances of achieving your desired weight and maintaining a healthier lifestyle.

Chapter 9: Setting Realistic Goals

Setting realistic goals is a fundamental and crucial aspect of achieving successful weight loss. Unrealistic goals can lead to frustration, discouragement, and even failure. In this note, we will explore the importance of setting realistic weight loss goals and provide guidance on how to establish them effectively.

Steps for Setting Realistic Weight Loss Goals:

Consider Your Starting Point: Your current weight, body composition, and activity level are important factors to consider when setting your goals. Set realistic expectations based on your current starting point.

Understand Healthy Weight Loss Rates: Aim for a weight loss rate of about 0.5 to 2 pounds (0.2 to 0.9 kilograms) per week. This rate is considered safe and sustainable.

Be Specific: Define your goals with clarity. Instead of saying, "I want to lose weight," specify the amount you wish to lose and the timeframe in which you want to achieve it.

Break Down Your Goals: Divide your overall weight loss goal into smaller, more manageable milestones. For example, if your ultimate goal is to lose 50 pounds, set milestones of 5 or 10 pounds along the way.

Focus on Behavior Changes: Place emphasis on behavior-based goals rather than solely on the number on the scale. For instance, set goals related to exercise frequency, daily calorie intake, or increased consumption of fruits and vegetables.

Use the SMART Framework: Apply the SMART (Specific, Measurable, Achievable, Relevant, Time-bound) framework to your goals. SMART goals are well-defined and actionable. For example, a SMART goal could be, "I will lose 10 pounds in the next 10 weeks by reducing my daily calorie intake to 1,800 calories and exercising for 30 minutes five days a week."

Regularly Review and Adjust: Periodically evaluate your progress and make adjustments to your goals as needed. If you're consistently losing weight more slowly than anticipated, be patient and consider extending your timeframe. If you're exceeding your goals, it may be appropriate to adjust them.

Seek Support and Accountability: Share your goals with a support system, such as friends, family, or a weight loss group. Having others who can encourage and hold you accountable can be immensely helpful.

Celebrate Achievements:

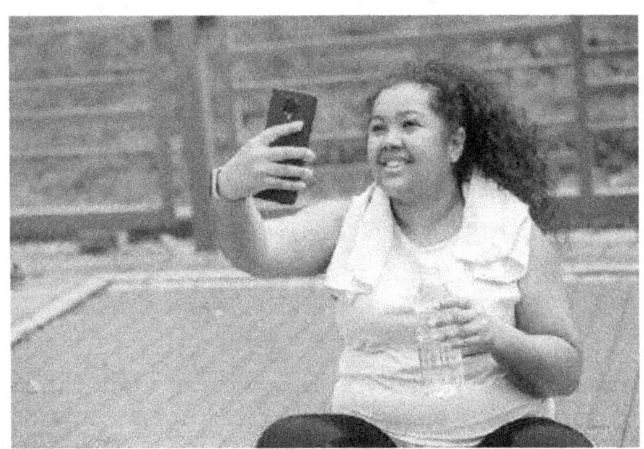

Acknowledge and cherish each accomplishment, regardless of its size. Acknowledging your accomplishments can help maintain motivation.

Evidently, setting realistic weight loss goals is a critical first step in your journey toward achieving a healthier body weight. Realistic goals provide motivation, support sustainability, promote a positive self-image, and contribute to overall well-being. By following the steps mentioned above and maintaining a balanced and gradual approach to weight loss, you can increase your chances of reaching your desired weight in a healthy and sustainable manner.

Chapter 10: Staying Consistent

Consistency is the key to achieving and maintaining weight loss. While embarking on a weight loss journey can be challenging, the results are highly rewarding. In this note, we will delve into the importance of consistency and explore practical strategies to help you stay on track throughout your weight loss journey.

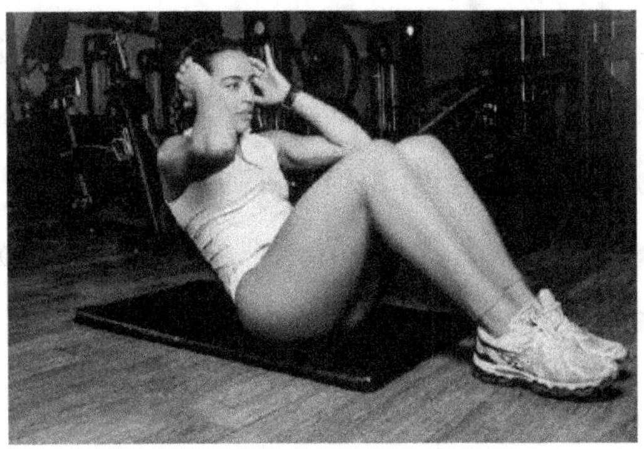

The Significance of Consistency:

Consistency is the backbone of successful weight loss. It involves sticking to your healthy habits and making them a regular part of your lifestyle. Here's why it's crucial:

Sustainable Progress: Consistency allows you to steadily progress towards your weight loss goals. Small, steady changes are more effective and sustainable than drastic, short-term measures.

Habit Formation: Consistency helps you establish healthy habits that become second nature over time. These habits are more likely to last and prevent weight regain.

Metabolism Stability: Maintaining consistent eating patterns and exercise routines helps regulate your metabolism, making it easier to manage your weight.

Psychological Benefits: Consistency fosters a sense of accomplishment and self-discipline, boosting your confidence and motivation.

Strategies for Staying Consistent:

1. Set Realistic Goals:

Start with achievable, specific, and time-bound goals. Unrealistic expectations can lead to frustration and a lack of consistency.

2. Create a Balanced Plan:

Opt for a balanced, sustainable approach to eating. Avoid extreme diets, as they are challenging to maintain in the long run.

3. Keep a Food Journal:

Monitoring daily consumption provides insights into eating habits, enabling necessary adjustments.

4. Regular Exercise:

Incorporate regular physical activity into your routine. Opt for enjoyable activities to boost the chances of maintaining consistency.

5. Meal Planning and Preparation:

Prearrange your meals and snacks to deter unplanned, unhealthy selections. This also helps you control portion sizes.

6. *Stay Hydrated*:

Adequate hydration is essential for weight management, as it curbs appetite and boosts metabolic processes.

7. *Seek Support*:

Discuss your objectives with a friend, family, or participate in a support network. Support and accountability can help you stay consistent.

8. *Mindful Eating*:

Engage in mindful eating by relishing every bite and being attuned to your body's hunger and fullness signals.

9. *Learn from Setbacks*:

Don't be discouraged by occasional setbacks. Use them as learning experiences to identify triggers and make necessary changes.

10. *Celebrate Milestones*:

Recognize and rejoice in your accomplishments, regardless of their size. Such positive reinforcement can enhance your motivation.

11. Prioritize Rest and Recovery:

Adequate sleep and rest are crucial for overall health and weight management. Ensure you get enough rest.

12. Stay Patient:

Understand that weight loss is a journey. Consistency doesn't always yield immediate results, but it's about long-term progress.

13. Professional Guidance:

Seek personalized advice and assistance from a healthcare provider or nutrition expert.

14. Positive Mindset:

Maintain a positive attitude throughout your journey. Self-belief and optimism play a significant role in consistency.

Consistency is the linchpin of successful weight loss. By setting realistic goals, creating sustainable habits, seeking support, and practicing healthy behaviors, you can maintain the consistency needed to achieve and maintain your weight loss goals. Remember, it's not about quick fixes but about making lasting, positive changes to your lifestyle for a healthier and happier you. Embrace the journey, stay consistent, and trust the process.

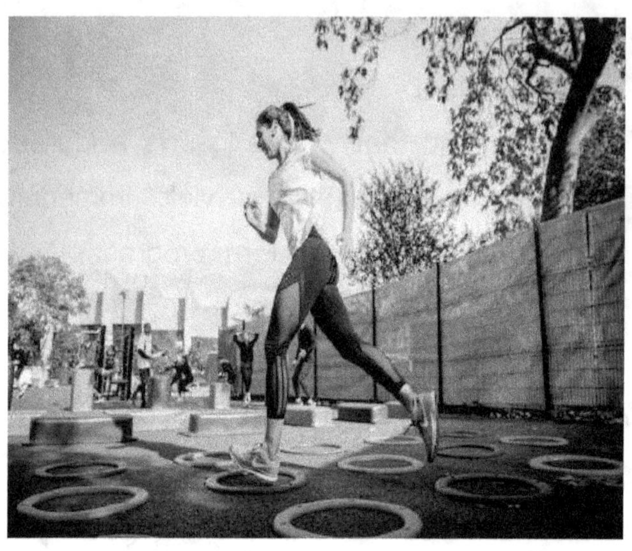

Chapter 11: Your New Life

Embarking on a weight loss journey is not just about shedding those extra pounds; it's a transformative experience that can have a profound impact on every aspect of your life. As you begin this incredible journey, here's a glimpse of what your new life might look like:

1. Improved Health: The most obvious benefit is improved health. You'll lower your risk of chronic diseases such as diabetes, heart disease, and high blood pressure. With a healthier weight, you're more likely to experience increased vitality and better overall well-being.

2. Boosted Confidence: Losing weight often leads to a surge in self-confidence. You'll feel better about your body, and this newfound confidence can spill over into your personal and professional life. You'll be more willing to take on challenges and embrace opportunities.

3. Renewed Energy: Say goodbye to sluggishness and fatigue. Weight loss brings an energy boost that allows you to be more active and engage in activities you might have avoided before. You'll find yourself exploring new hobbies and adventures with enthusiasm.

4. Improved Relationships: Weight loss can positively impact your relationships. Not only will you have more energy to spend quality time with loved ones, but your newfound confidence may also enhance your social interactions. It can lead to stronger bonds and a more active social life.

5. Better Sleep: Shedding excess weight can lead to better sleep. You'll experience fewer sleep disturbances and awaken feeling more refreshed. This improved sleep quality can significantly enhance your daily productivity and mood.

6. Healthier Eating Habits: As you work towards your weight loss goals, you'll likely adopt healthier eating habits. You'll become more mindful of what you consume, making better choices for your overall health. This shift can be a lifelong benefit.

7. Enhanced Mental Well-being: Weight loss can have a profound impact on your mental health. As you achieve your goals, you'll experience a sense of accomplishment and reduced stress. Regular exercise can release endorphins, which are natural mood lifters.

8. Wardrobe Makeover: A slimmer, healthier you will undoubtedly require a new wardrobe. Enjoy the process of shopping for clothes that you couldn't fit into before. The excitement of trying on smaller sizes is a significant motivational factor.

9. Newfound Discipline: Successful weight loss demands discipline, which can spill over into other areas of your life. You'll find that you're more determined and focused, making you better equipped to achieve other goals and tackle challenges.

10. Inspiration to Others: Your journey can inspire those around you. Friends and family may be motivated by your success to embark on their own path to a healthier life. Your dedication can have a ripple effect in your community.

Embarking on a weight loss journey is not just about the physical changes; it's a holistic transformation that touches every facet of your life. The benefits extend far beyond the number on the scale, giving you a new lease on life filled with improved health, confidence, and a fresh outlook on your future. Each step forward on this journey holds significant value and meaning.

•The Transformation: Real-Life Success Story of How Sarah Did It.

Sarah's ordeal began on a fateful night when she found herself gasping for breath, her heart racing uncontrollably. Rushed to the hospital, she was met with grim faces and unsettling statistics. The excessive weight gain had taken its toll, and she was at risk of losing not only her health but her life. It was the stark reality that shook her to her core.

In the dimly lit hospital room, the soft hum of machines was interrupted only by Sarah's shallow breaths. She lay surrounded by a labyrinth of tubes and monitors, an unsettling reminder of the weight that had nearly crushed her spirit. Sarah had reached a critical crossroads in her life, and the choices she made from that point would define her journey to recovery.

Amid the beeping machines and sterile hospital sheets, Sarah made a life-altering decision. She would choose life, no matter how hard the path to recovery might be. The journey from that hospital bed to a healthier version of herself was going to be arduous, but she was determined to persevere.

Her turning point arrived during a routine doctor's appointment. The scale displayed a number that shocked her and a stern warning from her physician about the health risks associated with her obesity. That day, she decided that enough was enough. She resolved to take control of her life and embarked on her weight loss journey.

Sarah knew that change would not come easy. She began by overhauling her eating habits. Out went the sugary snacks and fast food, and in came fresh fruits, vegetables, and lean proteins. She also committed to regular exercise, starting with gentle walks and gradually working her way up to more intense workouts. It was a challenging path, but she was determined to succeed.

The journey was fraught with hurdles, but Sarah celebrated every small victory along the way. Each pound lost and each milestone reached fueled her determination. She found support from friends, family, and even joined a local weight loss group, where she shared her challenges and learned from others' experiences.

Sarah's journey was not without setbacks. There were moments of self-doubt, cravings that seemed insurmountable, and days when the scale didn't budge. But she never gave up. She learned that setbacks were just temporary detours on the path to success.

As days turned into weeks, weeks into months, and months turned into years, Sarah's transformation became undeniable. Her smile, once hidden, was radiant. She had lost a significant amount of weight, but her gains extended far beyond the physical. Her confidence soared, and she radiated a positivity that inspired everyone around her.

Sarah's story began to inspire those in her community. She became an advocate for healthy living, sharing her journey on social media and speaking at local events. People from all walks of life found hope in her words and started their journeys towards healthier lives.

Years after that fateful doctor's appointment, Sarah had not only shed excess weight but had reclaimed her life. She was thriving, pursuing her passions, and helping others do the same. Her story was a testament to the incredible strength of the human spirit.

Sarah's remarkable journey from obesity to a healthier, happier life was a testament to the power of determination and resilience. A Triumph of the Human Spirit.

Her story shows that no matter how challenging the path, with unwavering commitment and a strong support system, one can triumph over adversity. Sarah's journey serves as an inspiration to anyone facing the daunting challenge of obesity, reminding them that transformation is possible and that a brighter, healthier future awaits.

MAN AND WOMAN FIT PROGRESS
vector icons

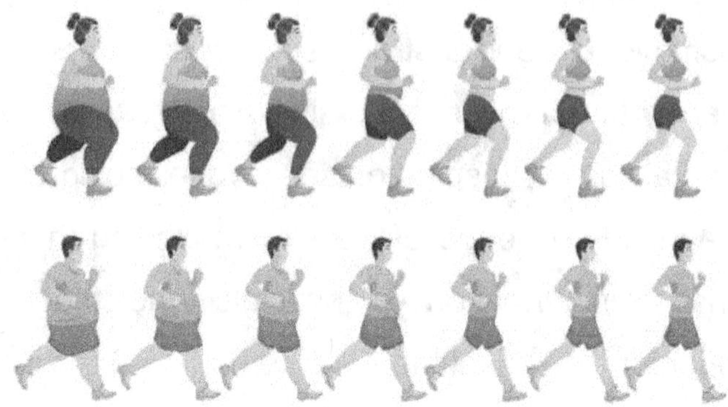

How to be a healthy woman?

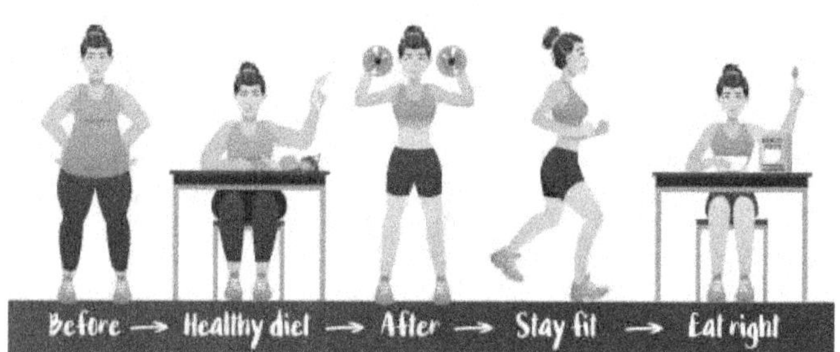

How to be a healthy man?

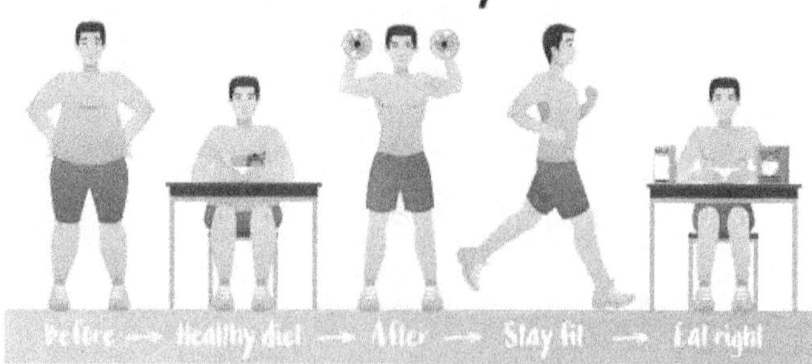

Conclusion

•Your Journey Begins Now

My dear friend, the journey of shedding weight and living a physically fit life is worth embarking on, as the benefits are immensely great and satisfying.

I understand that the journey can be challenging, even daunting at times. It's not just about losing pounds or gaining muscle; it's about taking control of your life, your health, and your happiness. But I promise you, the reward at the end of this path is worth every drop of sweat, every healthy meal, and every ounce of determination.

The first step on this journey is to believe in yourself. Believe you can do it! You possess incredible potential, and the power to change your life for the better is within you. The aim isn't perfection; it's about continuous progress.

Embrace your unique journey, with all its ups and downs, and use it to become the best version of yourself.

Build a network of supporters who share your ambitions; confide in friends, family, or connect with a community of like-minded people. You'll find strength in numbers, and together, you can inspire and uplift each other.

Set clear, achievable goals and celebrate every small victory along the way. Every pound lost, every extra mile run, and every new healthy habit adopted is a testament to your strength and determination. Celebrate these milestones, for they are the stepping stones to your success.

Remember, the journey to a physically fit life is not just about the body; it's about the mind too. Challenge your inner critic, replace self-doubt with self-belief, and use setbacks as stepping stones for growth. Embrace a positive mindset that reminds you that you are capable of achieving anything you set your mind to.

Consistency is key. There will be days when motivation wanes, and the path ahead seems long and uncertain. Recall your initial motivation during challenging moments. Visualize the healthier, happier, and more energetic version of yourself that you are striving to become. Use that vision as your guiding light.

Lastly, be patient with yourself. Transformation takes time. This is not a sprint; it's a marathon. The beauty of this journey is in its endurance, in the commitment you make to yourself every day.

So, I implore you to embark on this incredible journey to shed weight and live a physically fit life. Your health, your happiness, and your future self will thank you. Believe in yourself, find your support system, set goals, stay positive, be consistent, and be patient. Your journey is a story of strength, determination, and resilience. You possess greater potential than you can fathom. Embrace the process, and let it lead you to a healthier, happier, and more vibrant life.

Start today, and you'll be amazed at what you can achieve. Your journey begins now.

* 9 7 9 8 8 6 6 4 7 8 2 4 8 *